Neurogenic Communication Disorders: A Functional Approach